Shattering Stigma: A Comprehensive Guide from the Perspective of a Mental Health Specialist

About the author

Seán O'Connor is a passionate mental health advocate, author, and dedicated individual who has been actively involved in various aspects of the mental health field. With a wealth of experience as a layperson in mental health tribunals, counselling, coaching, and working in addiction with dual diagnosis, Sean brings a unique perspective to his ground-breaking book, "Shattering Stigma: A Comprehensive Guide."

Seán's journey began as a layperson, driven by a deep-rooted desire to contribute to the betterment of mental health services. Recognizing the importance of empowering individuals and advocating for their rights, he actively participates in mental health tribunals, gaining valuable insight into the challenges faced by those with mental health issues within the legal system. Through his involvement, Seán witnessed first-hand the need for comprehensive support and guidance for individuals navigating the complex landscape of mental health services.

Inspired by his experiences, Seán pursued additional training and education to further his understanding of mental health and support systems. Although not formally trained as a mental health professional, he dedicated himself to studying counselling techniques, coaching methodologies, and addiction treatment strategies.

His self-driven pursuit of knowledge, combined with his natural empathy and compassion, allowed him to effectively support individuals struggling with mental health and addiction.

Throughout his journey, Seán has worked alongside mental health professionals, providing invaluable insights from his layperson perspective. His collaborative approach, coupled with his dedication to learning and growth, has earned him the respect and trust of his colleagues and peers in the field.

"Shattering Stigma: A Comprehensive Guide" is the culmination of Seán's experiences, observations, and research. In this transformative book, he presents a comprehensive understanding of mental health challenges, addiction, and the intertwining nature of dual diagnosis. Drawing on his experiences as a layperson and his interactions with mental health professionals, Sean offers practical advice, actionable strategies, and an empathetic perspective to help individuals facing mental health issues navigate their journeys to recovery.

Beyond his work as an author, Seán actively engages with the mental health community through public speaking engagements, workshops, and advocacy efforts. By openly sharing his experiences and insights, he seeks to challenge societal stigmas, foster understanding, and encourage empathy towards individuals struggling with mental health challenges.

Seán O'Connor's dedication to mental health advocacy is rooted in his unwavering belief that every individual deserves access to compassionate and effective support. His book, "Shattering Stigma: A Comprehensive Guide," serves as a testament to his commitment to empowering others, offering practical guidance, and promoting awareness. Through his unique perspective as a layperson, Seán inspires hope, instils resilience, and catalyses positive change in the lives of those facing mental health challenges

Career background

Seán O'Connor is a highly accomplished health professional with a diverse range of experiences and a strong commitment to making a positive impact in the field of health and well-being. Currently serving as a Project Manager in Arts & Health within the Health Service Executive (HSE), Seán is dedicated to exploring the intersections between creativity and health to enhance the well-being of individuals and staff.

In addition to his role in Arts & Health, Seán holds a significant position as a lay member on tribunal panels for the Mental Health Commission. This involvement allows him to contribute to the fair and just assessment of mental health cases, ensuring that the rights and well-being of individuals are protected.

Seán is also deeply passionate about road safety and has developed the Drive Aware Programme (DAP) as a means to effect positive changes in attitudes and behaviours related to impaired, dangerous, and careless driving. Through his program, Seán aims to promote responsible driving practices and reduce the risks associated with reckless behaviour on the roads. His dedication to enhancing road safety has led him to deliver the Drive Aware Programme throughout the country.

As the founder of Seán O'Connor Coaching, Seán offers personalized one-on-one coaching sessions and conducts training workshops and seminars. Leveraging his extensive knowledge and experience, he empowers individuals to overcome challenges, improve their well-being, and achieve personal and professional growth.

Throughout his career, Seán has held various impactful positions. He served as a Project Manager with the HSE National Clinical Programme for People with Disability, where he played a pivotal role in improving healthcare services and support for individuals with disabilities.

As a Task Force Manager in the HSE Drugs & Alcohol sector, Seán contributed to the development and implementation of strategies to address substance abuse issues within the community.

His previous roles also include serving as the Director of the Dyslexia Association of Ireland, where he championed the rights and needs of individuals with dyslexia, and as the Chairperson and Director of Pieta House, an organization dedicated to preventing suicide and providing support to those in crisis.

Furthermore,

Seán has a unique background in the legal field, having served as a sitting Magistrate/Justice of the Peace within Her Majesty's Court Service. He brings a profound understanding of the criminal justice system and leverages this knowledge to make fair and informed decisions.

Seán 's expertise extends to the field of addiction counselling, having worked as an Addiction Counsellor in both community and prison settings. He has provided vital support and guidance to individuals struggling with addiction, helping them on their journey towards recovery. Seán has also contributed to the provision of counselling services within the prison setting, recognizing the importance of addressing mental health needs in such environments.

Additionally, Seán has made valuable contributions to the criminal justice system as a Drug & Alcohol worker with Probation Services. His work in this capacity focused on assisting individuals in overcoming addiction, reintegrating into society, and reducing reoffending rates.

Media work within TV and radio has provided Seán with a platform to raise awareness about various health and social issues. He has utilized these mediums to educate and inform the public, advocating for positive change and promoting well-being.

Seán 's career began in engineering, where he embarked on a four-year apprenticeship as a fresh-faced sixteen-year-old. He gained invaluable experience working for a large multinational Oil and Gas company, further developing his skills and contributing to the industry.

With an impressive array of experiences spanning healthcare, project management, coaching, counselling, advocacy, and engineering, Seán O'Connor embodies a passionate and dedicated health professional committed to improving the lives of individuals and communities.

His multifaceted background and expertise enable him to address complex challenges, inspire positive change, and empower others to reach their full potential.

And for further insights into Sean's career to date please visit LinkedIn

https://www.linkedin.com/in/sean-oconnor/

Here's a quick rundown of Seán's publications to date:

A Therapist's Guide to a Little Bit of Everything: is a comprehensive and invaluable resource designed to support therapists in navigating a wide range of topics and issues they may encounter in their practice.

Leading in Healthcare Management and Leadership in the UK and Ireland - Exploring the intricacies of healthcare leadership and management, shedding light on effective practices in this ever-evolving field.

Leading with Purpose: A Guide to Being an Effective Chairperson in the Charity Sector of the UK and Ireland - Offering guidance to aspiring and current chairpersons, emphasizing the importance of purpose-driven leadership in the non-profit sector.

Breaking the Chains: A Comprehensive Guide to Addiction Counselling in Ireland and the UK' - Shedding light on effective counselling techniques and strategies to support individuals in overcoming addiction.

Empowering Voices: A Comprehensive Guide to Becoming a Freelance Contributor in Drug and Alcohol Addiction Journalism - A resource for aspiring freelance journalists interested in covering the crucial topics of drug and alcohol addiction.

Drive Aware: "Safer roads for a safer society" - This has been the driving principle behind the ambitious initiative known as the Drive Aware program in Ireland.

Empowering Change: A Project Manager's Perspective on the Disability Sector in Ireland: This comprehensive induction provides you with a strong foundation to navigate your role as a Project Manager in the disability sector.

Balancing Justice: A Magistrate's Journey - Sharing my personal experiences and insights as a magistrate, highlighting the challenges and rewards of serving in the legal system.

Mastering Life Coaching: A Comprehensive Guide for Professional Coaches - Equipping life coaches with the necessary tools and knowledge to empower their clients and facilitate positive change.

Clearing the Air: Smoking Cessation Services in the UK and their Benefits to Society - Advocating for the importance of smoking cessation and exploring the valuable services available to individuals looking to quit smoking.

Engineering Excellence: Unveiling the Potential of the Gas and Petroleum Industry' - An exploration of the gas and petroleum industry, revealing the incredible potential and advancements within this vital sector.

Plumbing for beginners: A Guide for Plumbers in the UK and Ireland. This book is specifically designed to provide aspiring plumbers, and plumbing enthusiasts in the United Kingdom and Ireland.

All of the above publications can be found at

https://www.amazon.co.uk/~/e/B0C8G4ZN94

Where you can contact him

Seán O'Connor Coaching

https://www.seanoconnorcoaching.com/

Drive Aware Ireland

https://www.driveaware.ie/

Table of Contents

Chapter 11: Legal Framework and Key Legislation

Chapter 12: The Importance of Laypersons in Tribunal Panels

Chapter 13: Ethical Considerations and Confidentiality

Chapter 14: The Layperson's Role

14.1 Qualities and Skills of an Effective Lay Advocate

14.2 Identifying the essential qualities and skills required for effective advocacy.

14.3 Active listening, empathy, and effective communication techniques.

14.4 Developing a non-judgmental and compassionate approach.

Chapter 15: Working Collaboratively with Healthcare Professionals

15.1 Establishing collaborative relationships with psychiatrists, nurses, and other professionals.

15.2 Understanding their perspectives while maintaining an independent role.

15.3 Effective communication strategies for interdisciplinary collaboration.

Chapter 16: Cultural Sensitivity and Diversity Awareness

16.1 Recognizing the importance of cultural sensitivity in mental health advocacy.

16.2 Understanding the impact of cultural and social factors on patients' experiences.

16.3 Respecting and accommodating diverse backgrounds, beliefs, and practices.

Chapter 17: Confidentiality and Maintaining Boundaries

17.1 Understanding the legal and ethical obligations of maintaining patient confidentiality.

17.2 Establishing clear boundaries in interactions with patients and healthcare professionals.

17.3 Safeguarding patient information and records.

Chapter 18: Building Rapport and Effective Communication

18.1 Strategies for building trust and rapport with patients during tribunal proceedings.

18.2 Effective communication techniques, including active listening and clear explanations.

18.3 Addressing language barriers and ensuring effective communication with diverse populations.

Chapter 19: Conclusion

19.1 Recap of key findings and recommendations

19.2 The collective responsibility towards mental health

19.3 Fostering hope and recovery

19.4 Inspiring a mentally healthy Ireland

Introduction: Shattering Stigma

Mental health services in Ireland are crucial for addressing the psychological well-being of individuals and promoting their overall quality of life. As a mental health specialist, your expertise and insights play a vital role in understanding and providing effective care within this context. This book aims to provide you with an in-depth exploration of mental health services in Ireland, offering a comprehensive understanding of the field from your unique perspective.

Through detailed chapters, we will examine various aspects of mental health services, including assessment, diagnosis, treatment approaches, specialized services, community-based care, challenges, and opportunities.

Within the confines of Irish society, mental health has long been overshadowed by stigma and misconceptions. Generations have suffered silently, their anguish hidden behind closed doors. However, the tides are turning, and a collective awakening is occurring.

Today, mental health is recognized as a fundamental aspect of overall well-being, and Ireland is embracing the imperative of providing quality mental health services to its citizens.

The importance of mental health services in Ireland cannot be overstated. Mental health disorders affect individuals of all ages, genders, and backgrounds, permeating every aspect of their lives. They impact families, communities, and society as a whole. Recognizing the profound societal impact of mental health, Ireland has committed to strengthening its mental health services, striving to create a support system that promotes recovery, resilience, and hope.

Addressing the prevailing stigma surrounding mental health is paramount in this endeavour. For far too long, individuals grappling with mental health challenges have faced discrimination, judgment, and isolation.

Yet, we know that mental health disorders are not a reflection of personal weakness or character flaws; they are genuine health conditions that require understanding, empathy, and effective interventions. As mental health specialists, we have a crucial role to play in dismantling these barriers, challenging societal attitudes, and fostering an environment of acceptance and compassion.

This book aims to provide a comprehensive exploration of mental health services in Ireland, looking into the intricacies of assessment, diagnosis, and treatment. It will examine the evolution of mental health services, from the historical context to the current legislative and policy frameworks.

We will explore the diverse array of specialized services available, focusing on child and adolescent mental health, adult mental health, geriatric mental health, and addiction and substance abuse services. Additionally, we will delve into the crucial role of community-based care and the invaluable support services that bolster mental health resilience within local communities.

While progress has been made, challenges remain. Workforce shortages, limited resources, and ongoing stigma pose significant obstacles to the provision of comprehensive and accessible mental health care. Through this book, we will examine these challenges and explore potential solutions, addressing the need for increased funding, policy reform, and innovative approaches. It is our collective responsibility to advocate for a robust mental health system that empowers individuals, families, and communities to thrive.

As mental health specialists, we are not merely observers of the mental health landscape; we are catalysts for change. Our professional development, self-care, and collaboration are essential for delivering the highest standard of care to those in need.

We will explore opportunities for advocacy, networking, and driving policy reform, aiming to create a future where mental health is prioritized, stigma is eradicated, and hope flourishes.

Together, let us embark on a transformative journey through the realms of mental health services in Ireland. With each page turned, we will deepen our understanding, challenge our assumptions, and foster a society where every individual feels supported, valued, and empowered. Together, we can shatter the stigma surrounding mental health and nurture a mentally healthy Ireland.

Chapter 1: Understanding Mental Health in Ireland

1.1 Overview of Mental Health and Its Impact

Mental health is an integral component of overall well-being, encompassing emotional, psychological, and social aspects of our lives.

In Ireland, as in any other nation, mental health profoundly affects individuals, families, communities, and society as a whole. Understanding the impact of mental health disorders is crucial for comprehending the significance of mental health services in Ireland.

Mental health disorders are diverse in nature, ranging from mood disorders like depression and bipolar disorder to anxiety disorders, schizophrenia, and personality disorders. These conditions can impair an individual's ability to cope with daily challenges, maintain relationships, and pursue their goals and aspirations.

They may also contribute to a higher risk of physical health problems and a reduced quality of life.

1.2 Historical Context of Mental Health in Ireland

To understand the current state of mental health services in Ireland, it is important to consider the historical context. Historically, Ireland, like many other countries, has grappled with a legacy of institutionalization and stigma surrounding mental health. The widespread practice of institutionalizing individuals with mental health conditions led to their exclusion from society, perpetuating a cycle of isolation, neglect, and mistreatment.

However, significant progress has been made in recent decades. Ireland has witnessed a shift toward community-based care, the deinstitutionalization of mental health services, and a recognition of the importance of human rights and dignity for individuals with mental health challenges.

1.3 Prevalence and Types of Mental Health Disorders in Ireland

Mental health disorders are prevalent in Ireland, affecting people of all ages and backgrounds.

According to the National Survey of Psychiatric Morbidity in Ireland, conducted in 2012, approximately one in seven adults in Ireland reported experiencing a mental health disorder in the previous year. This prevalence underscores the urgent need for accessible and effective mental health services across the country.

Common mental health disorders in Ireland include depression, anxiety disorders, substance abuse disorders, and bipolar disorder. The impact of these conditions extends beyond the individual, affecting families, workplaces, and communities. It is essential to recognize the diverse manifestations of mental health disorders and the unique challenges they present to individuals seeking support.

1.4 Sociocultural Factors Influencing Mental Health

The mental health of individuals is influenced by a complex interplay of sociocultural factors. Ireland's social, economic, and cultural context shapes the experiences and perceptions of mental health within the population. Factors such as poverty, unemployment, social isolation, discrimination, and migration can contribute to the development and exacerbation of mental health disorders.

The legacy of cultural attitudes and beliefs surrounding mental health also plays a role. Stigma, shame, and a lack of understanding can hinder individuals from seeking help or disclosing their struggles. However, Ireland has witnessed a gradual shift in attitudes, with increased awareness and efforts to reduce stigma and promote mental health literacy.

Understanding the sociocultural factors that influence mental health is crucial for tailoring mental health services to the unique needs of the Irish population. By acknowledging the diverse challenges faced by individuals and communities, mental health specialists can provide more inclusive and effective support.

In Chapter 1, we have explored the fundamental aspects of mental health in Ireland. We have gained an understanding of the impact of mental health disorders, examined the historical context, explored the prevalence of mental health disorders, and considered the sociocultural factors that shape mental health experiences. By delving into these foundational elements, we are better equipped to comprehend the importance and relevance of mental health services in Ireland. In the subsequent chapters, we will delve deeper into the structure, challenges, and opportunities within the mental health system, with a focus on assessment, treatment, specialized services, and community-based care.

Chapter 2: Mental Health Services in Ireland: An Overview

2.1 Evolution of Mental Health Services

The provision of mental health services in Ireland has undergone significant changes over the years. Historically, mental health care was predominantly centered around large institutions, often characterized by a custodial approach that lacked a focus on individualized care and recovery.

However, following a wave of deinstitutionalization and a growing understanding of community-based care, Ireland has embraced a more person-centered and community-oriented approach to mental health services.

In recent decades, there has been a shift towards developing a comprehensive mental health system that promotes recovery, early intervention, and integration with primary care services. This evolution reflects a recognition of the importance of providing accessible and holistic mental health care to all individuals in need.

2.2 Legislation and Policies Governing Mental Health Services

The provision of mental health services in Ireland is guided by a framework of legislation and policies aimed at protecting the rights and well-being of individuals with mental health challenges. The Mental Health Act 2001 is a crucial legislative piece that provides a legal framework for the care and treatment of individuals with mental health disorders. It emphasizes the principles of least restrictive care, informed consent, and the rights of individuals to participate in decisions about their treatment.

In addition to legislation, several policy documents and strategic plans have shaped the landscape of mental health services in Ireland. The "A Vision for Change" policy, published in 2006, is a landmark document that outlines a blueprint for the development of mental health services, focusing on recovery, community-based care, and the integration of mental health into primary care settings.

Other policy initiatives, such as the "Connecting for Life" strategy, have been instrumental in addressing the issue of suicide prevention in Ireland.

2.3 Structure and Organization of Mental Health Services

The mental health service delivery system in Ireland is structured to cater to the diverse needs of the population. Mental health services are provided through a combination of statutory, voluntary, and private organizations.

At the national level, the Health Service Executive (HSE) plays a crucial role in the planning, funding, and coordination of mental health services. The HSE oversees the operation of mental health teams, including community mental health teams and specialist services, which are responsible for providing assessment, treatment, and support to individuals with mental health disorders.

Primary care services, including general practitioners (GPs) and primary care mental health teams, form an essential part of the mental health system. They provide initial assessments, treatment, and referrals, serving as a gateway to specialized mental health services.

Voluntary and non-governmental organizations (NGOs) also contribute significantly to the provision of mental health services in Ireland. These organizations offer a range of supports, including advocacy, counselling, helplines, and community-based programs.

2.4 Role of Different Stakeholders

Mental health services in Ireland involve the collaboration of various stakeholders, each playing a crucial role in the delivery and improvement of services.

These stakeholders include government bodies, mental health professionals, service users and their families, NGOs, and the broader community.

The government, through its policies, legislation, and funding, shapes the overall direction and priorities of mental health services. Mental health professionals, including psychiatrists, psychologists, nurses, social workers, and occupational therapists, provide assessment, diagnosis, treatment, and support to individuals with mental health challenges.

Service users and their families have an active role in the development and evaluation of mental health services, advocating for their needs, and sharing their experiences to drive positive change. NGOs and community organizations contribute to mental health promotion, awareness, and support, often filling gaps in service provision and providing invaluable resources to the community.

2.5 The Way Forward: Challenges and Opportunities

While Ireland has made significant progress in the provision of mental health services, challenges remain. Workforce shortages, limited resources, long waiting lists, and regional disparities in access to services continue to be major obstacles.

Additionally, stigma and discrimination surrounding mental health persist, hindering help-seeking behaviour and social inclusion.

However, amidst these challenges lie opportunities for improvement. Increased investment in mental health services, including staffing, infrastructure, and community supports, is crucial for meeting the growing demand. Strengthening the integration of mental health with primary care services can enhance early intervention and ensure a more coordinated and holistic approach to care.

Advancements in technology, such as tele psychiatry and digital mental health interventions, offer innovative avenues for expanding access to care and supporting individuals remotely. Furthermore, ongoing efforts to reduce stigma, promote mental health literacy, and foster a culture of open dialogue are key in transforming the mental health landscape in Ireland.

In Chapter 2, we have explored the overview of mental health services in Ireland. We have traced the evolution of these services, examined the legislation and policies that govern them, and outlined the structure and organization of the mental health system. By understanding the role of different stakeholders and recognizing the challenges and opportunities that lie ahead, we lay the foundation for a deeper exploration of assessment, treatment approaches, specialized services, and community-based care in the subsequent chapters.

Chapter 3: Assessing and Diagnosing Mental Health Disorders

3.1 The Importance of Assessment and Diagnosis

Accurate assessment and diagnosis form the cornerstone of effective mental health care.

They provide a framework for understanding an individual's presenting symptoms, formulating an appropriate treatment plan, and monitoring progress over time.

In Ireland, mental health professionals employ a comprehensive approach to assessment and diagnosis, considering various factors to ensure a holistic understanding of the individual's mental health.

3.2 Multidimensional Assessment

Assessing mental health involves a multidimensional evaluation that encompasses different aspects of an individual's life. This includes gathering information about their medical history, current symptoms, psychosocial context, and functional impairments. Mental health professionals utilize various assessment tools, interviews, and observation to obtain a comprehensive understanding of the individual's mental health status.

Psychological assessments, such as interviews and questionnaires, help gather subjective information about the individual's thoughts, feelings, and behaviours.

They aid in identifying the presence of specific mental health disorders, assessing symptom severity, and monitoring treatment progress. Additionally, collateral information from family members, caregivers, or other relevant sources may provide valuable insights into the individual's functioning.

3.3 Diagnostic Classification Systems

In Ireland, mental health disorders are diagnosed using widely accepted diagnostic classification systems, such as the Diagnostic and Statistical Manual of Mental Disorders (DSM) and the International Classification of Diseases (ICD). These systems provide a standardized set of diagnostic criteria and classification guidelines that help mental health professionals classify and describe different mental health disorders.

The DSM, published by the American Psychiatric Association, is commonly used in Ireland and provides a comprehensive framework for diagnosing mental health disorders. It classifies disorders into specific categories based on symptom presentation and duration. The ICD, developed by the World Health Organization (WHO), is used globally and includes both physical and mental health disorders. It provides a broader perspective on mental health disorders and incorporates a biopsychosocial approach to diagnosis.

3.4 Cultural Considerations in Assessment and Diagnosis

Cultural factors significantly influence how mental health is experienced, expressed, and perceived.

In Ireland, mental health professionals recognize the importance of cultural sensitivity and competence in assessment and diagnosis. They consider the cultural background, beliefs, and values of the individual when interpreting symptoms and formulating a diagnosis.

Culturally appropriate assessment tools and techniques are employed to ensure that the assessment process respects and accommodates diverse cultural perspectives. Mental health professionals strive to develop a collaborative and respectful relationship with individuals from different cultural backgrounds, fostering an environment where they feel comfortable discussing their mental health concerns.

3.5 Challenges and Limitations in Assessment and Diagnosis

Assessing and diagnosing mental health disorders can present challenges and limitations. Subjective reporting, cultural and linguistic barriers, and the complex nature of mental health symptoms can impact the accuracy and reliability of assessments.

Additionally, comorbidity (the presence of multiple mental health disorders) and the overlap of symptoms across different disorders can pose diagnostic challenges.

Furthermore, mental health assessments are dynamic processes, and symptoms may fluctuate over time. Regular reassessment and ongoing monitoring are necessary to capture changes in symptoms, treatment response, and overall functioning.

In Chapter 3, we have explored the critical process of assessing and diagnosing mental health disorders in Ireland. We have highlighted the multidimensional nature of assessments, the use of diagnostic classification systems, and the significance of cultural considerations.

We have also acknowledged the challenges and limitations in the assessment process. In the subsequent chapters, we will delve deeper into evidence-based treatment approaches, specialized services, and community-based care, aiming to provide a comprehensive understanding of mental health services in Ireland.

Chapter 4: Treatment Approaches in Mental Health Services

4.1 The Multimodal Nature of Mental Health Treatment

Treatment approaches in mental health services encompass a range of interventions aimed at promoting recovery, managing symptoms, and improving overall well-being. These approaches recognize the multidimensional nature of mental health and address the biological, psychological, and social aspects of individuals' lives.

In Ireland, mental health professionals employ a diverse array of evidence-based treatment approaches to meet the unique needs of individuals with mental health disorders.

4.2 Medication-Based Interventions

Medication-based interventions, such as psychotropic medications, play a crucial role in the treatment of many mental health disorders.

Psychiatrists and other healthcare professionals with prescribing authority carefully evaluate individuals and prescribe appropriate medications based on diagnosis, symptom severity, and individual response.

Psychotropic medications include antidepressants, antipsychotics, mood stabilizers, and anxiolytics. These medications help manage symptoms, alleviate distress, and restore the chemical imbalances that contribute to mental health disorders. Regular monitoring, dosage adjustments, and ongoing communication between the individual and their healthcare provider are essential for optimizing medication efficacy and minimizing side effects.

4.3 Psychotherapy and Counselling

Psychotherapy and counselling are integral components of mental health treatment. These approaches involve therapeutic interactions between mental health professionals and individuals with mental health disorders, focusing on exploring emotions, thoughts, and behaviours to promote insight, coping skills, and personal growth.

Various types of psychotherapy are utilized in Ireland, including cognitive-behavioural therapy (CBT), psychodynamic therapy, interpersonal therapy, and mindfulness-based approaches. CBT, in particular, is widely used and emphasizes the connection between thoughts, emotions, and behaviours, helping individuals develop adaptive coping strategies and challenge maladaptive patterns.

Counselling, which may be provided by psychologists, counsellors, or social workers, offers supportive and non-directive interventions, helping individuals explore their concerns, gain perspective, and develop strategies to navigate challenges.

It can be particularly beneficial in addressing issues such as grief, relationship difficulties, and life transitions.

4.4 Rehabilitation and Recovery-Oriented Interventions

Rehabilitation and recovery-oriented interventions aim to support individuals in regaining and maintaining functional independence and overall well-being. These interventions recognize that mental health recovery is a personal journey that goes beyond symptom reduction and encompasses aspects of empowerment, self-determination, and community integration.

Rehabilitation programs may include vocational training, educational support, social skills development, and assistance with daily living activities. They promote the individual's ability to participate in meaningful activities, enhance social connections, and build a sense of purpose and identity beyond their mental health condition.

Recovery-oriented approaches emphasize collaboration between individuals, mental health professionals, and support networks. They focus on the individual's strengths, resilience, and goals, empowering them to take an active role in their recovery process. Peer support, self-help groups, and recovery-focused workshops are essential components of these interventions, fostering a sense of belonging, hope, and mutual understanding.

4.5 Integrative and Holistic Care

In Ireland, there is increasing recognition of the importance of integrative and holistic care approaches in mental health services.

These approaches acknowledge that mental health disorders are complex and require a comprehensive understanding of an individual's physical, psychological, and social well-being.

Integrative care involves collaboration between mental health professionals and other healthcare providers, such as primary care physicians, to address both mental and physical health needs. This approach ensures coordinated and holistic care, considering the interconnectedness of mental and physical well-being.

Holistic care emphasizes the promotion of overall well-being by incorporating complementary therapies, lifestyle changes, and self-care practices. These may include exercise, nutrition, mindfulness, relaxation techniques, and complementary therapies like art therapy or music therapy. Holistic care aims to enhance individuals' self-awareness, self-management, and resilience.

4.6 The Importance of Individualized Treatment Planning

In Ireland, mental health professionals recognize the significance of individualized treatment planning. Each person's mental health journey is unique, and treatment approaches should be tailored to their specific needs, preferences, and circumstances.

Collaboration and shared decision-making between individuals and mental health professionals are essential to develop personalized treatment plans.

Individualized treatment planning involves considering factors such as cultural background, age, gender, and personal goals.

It takes into account the individual's strengths, challenges, and support systems, ensuring that the treatment approach aligns with their values and promotes their overall well-being.

In Chapter 4, we have explored the various treatment approaches used in mental health services in Ireland. From medication-based interventions to psychotherapy, rehabilitation, and integrative care, these approaches reflect the comprehensive and person-centered nature of mental health care. Recognizing the importance of individualized treatment planning, we aim to empower individuals on their recovery journey and improve their quality of life. In the following chapters, we will delve into specialized mental health services and the integration of care within the community context.

Chapter 5: Specialized Mental Health Services in Ireland

5.1 Introduction to Specialized Mental Health Services

In Ireland, specialized mental health services cater to specific populations or address particular mental health needs.

These services are designed to provide targeted and specialized care, ensuring that individuals receive appropriate interventions and support tailored to their unique circumstances. This chapter explores some of the key specialized mental health services available in Ireland.

5.2 Child and Adolescent Mental Health Services (CAMHS)

Child and Adolescent Mental Health Services (CAMHS) focus on the mental health needs of children and young people up to the age of 18.

CAMHS provide assessment, diagnosis, treatment, and support for a wide range of mental health disorders specific to this age group, such as anxiety, depression, attention-deficit hyperactivity disorder (ADHD), and eating disorders.

CAMHS teams typically include child psychiatrists, psychologists, nurses, social workers, and occupational therapists. They employ a range of interventions, including individual therapy, family therapy, play therapy, and medication management when necessary. Early intervention, prevention programs, and community outreach initiatives are key components of CAMHS to promote positive mental health in children and young people.

5.3 Adult Community Mental Health Services

Adult Community Mental Health Services focus on the mental health needs of adults aged 18 and above within the community setting.

These services aim to provide accessible, person-centered care to individuals with mental health disorders, promoting recovery, and supporting individuals to live fulfilling lives in their communities.

Community mental health teams typically consist of psychiatrists, psychologists, nurses, social workers, occupational therapists, and other mental health professionals. They offer a range of interventions, including assessment, treatment, crisis intervention, psychotherapy, and rehabilitation support.

Community-based services play a vital role in preventing hospitalization, promoting social inclusion, and facilitating individuals' integration into their communities.

5.4 Psychiatric Hospitals and Inpatient Services

Psychiatric hospitals and inpatient services are specialized facilities that provide acute care and treatment for individuals with severe mental health disorders. These services are designed for individuals who require intensive interventions, observation, and stabilization in a hospital setting.

Psychiatric hospitals have multidisciplinary teams that include psychiatrists, nurses, psychologists, social workers, and occupational therapists. They offer 24/7 care, ensuring the safety and well-being of individuals in crisis.

Treatment in psychiatric hospitals may include medication management, therapy, group activities, and discharge planning to facilitate a smooth transition back to the community.

5.5 Substance Abuse and Addiction Services

Substance abuse and addiction services address the complex needs of individuals struggling with substance use disorders. These services aim to provide integrated care, addressing both the mental health and addiction aspects of individuals' well-being.

Specialized addiction services in Ireland include outpatient clinics, detoxification units, residential rehabilitation centres, and harm reduction programs.

They offer a range of interventions, such as counselling, medication-assisted treatment, group therapy, relapse prevention, and aftercare support. Collaboration between mental health services, addiction services, and community supports is crucial to provide holistic care for individuals with co-occurring mental health and substance use disorders.

5.6 Geriatric Mental Health Services

Geriatric mental health services focus on the mental health needs of older adults. As the population ages, the demand for specialized mental health services for older adults has increased. These services address age-related mental health conditions, including dementia, depression, anxiety, and cognitive impairments.

Geriatric mental health teams typically include geriatric psychiatrists, psychologists, nurses, and occupational therapists. They provide comprehensive assessments, diagnosis, treatment, and support tailored to the unique needs of older adults.

Services may include memory clinics, day hospitals, community outreach, and support for family caregivers. The aim is to promote mental well-being, enhance quality of life, and support individuals in aging with dignity.

5.7 Forensic Mental Health Services

Forensic mental health services are specialized services that address the mental health needs of individuals involved in the criminal justice system.

These services focus on assessment, treatment, and risk management for individuals with mental health disorders who are in contact with the legal system.

Forensic mental health teams consist of forensic psychiatrists, psychologists, social workers, and other professionals with expertise in the intersection of mental health and the law. They provide assessment for fitness to stand trial, risk assessments, therapeutic interventions, and support for individuals transitioning back into the community after involvement with the criminal justice system. Collaboration between mental health services, legal professionals, and probation services is crucial to ensure comprehensive care and rehabilitation.

5.8 The Mental Health Commission

The Mental Health Commission in Ireland plays a vital role in overseeing and regulating mental health services to ensure the highest standards of care and protection for individuals experiencing mental health challenges.

As an independent statutory body, the Commission functions as an authoritative voice in the mental health sector, working collaboratively with various stakeholders including healthcare providers, policymakers, and service users. The Commission's responsibilities encompass monitoring and inspecting mental health services, promoting quality improvement initiatives, enforcing regulatory compliance, and advocating for the rights and well-being of patients. By establishing standards, conducting inspections, and offering guidance, the Mental Health Commission aims to create a more transparent, accountable, and person-centered mental health system in Ireland.

In Chapter 5, we have explored some of the key specialized mental health services in Ireland. These services cater to specific populations and address diverse mental health needs, recognizing the importance of tailored care and support. By providing specialized interventions, Ireland's mental health system aims to enhance the well-being and recovery of individuals across different stages of life and specific circumstances. In the subsequent chapter, we will examine the integration of mental health services within the community context, promoting accessibility, continuity of care, and social inclusion.

Chapter 6: Community-Based Mental Health Care

6.1 The Importance of Community-Based Mental Health Care

Community-based mental health care plays a vital role in promoting accessibility, continuity of care, and social inclusion for individuals with mental health disorders. This approach recognizes that mental health is influenced by various social determinants and that providing support within the community setting can have significant benefits for individuals' recovery and overall well-being. In Ireland, community-based mental health care is a key component of the mental health service delivery system.

6.2 Primary Care and Mental Health Integration

Integration of mental health care with primary care services is a fundamental aspect of community-based mental health care.

Primary care physicians, such as general practitioners (GPs), are often the first point of contact for individuals seeking help for mental health concerns. They play a crucial role in the early identification, assessment, and basic treatment of mental health disorders.

In Ireland, initiatives have been implemented to enhance the integration of mental health care into primary care settings. Collaborative care models, where mental health professionals work alongside GPs to provide comprehensive care, have been successful in improving access to mental health services and delivering more holistic care.

6.3 Community Mental Health Teams

Community mental health teams are interdisciplinary teams consisting of psychiatrists, psychologists, nurses, social workers, occupational therapists, and other professionals. These teams provide mental health care and support to individuals within the community setting.

Community mental health teams offer a range of services, including assessment, treatment, case management, and psychosocial interventions. They provide support for individuals with severe and enduring mental health disorders, helping them maintain stability, access necessary resources, and engage in meaningful activities. These teams also collaborate with other community services, such as housing agencies, employment support, and peer support networks, to address the broader social determinants of mental health.

6.4 Home-Based and Outreach Services

Home-based and outreach services are essential components of community-based mental health care. These services recognize that some individuals may face barriers in accessing traditional mental health services or may require more intensive support in their own environment.

Home-based services involve mental health professionals visiting individuals in their homes to provide assessment, treatment, and support. This approach enables a more personalized and supportive interaction, taking into account the individual's living conditions, family dynamics, and daily challenges.

Outreach services extend mental health care beyond the clinical setting, reaching individuals in community centres, shelters, schools, and other community locations. These services aim to improve accessibility, reduce stigma, and engage individuals who may not typically seek help.

6.5 Peer Support and Self-Help Groups

Peer support and self-help groups are integral to community-based mental health care. These groups provide individuals with lived experiences of mental health challenges an opportunity to connect, share experiences, and support one another in their recovery journeys.

Peer support programs are facilitated by trained individuals who have personal experience with mental health challenges. They provide empathy, understanding, and practical guidance to individuals who may feel more comfortable seeking support from peers.

Self-help groups, on the other hand, are facilitated by professionals or trained volunteers and offer a structured space for individuals to discuss common challenges, learn coping strategies, and develop a sense of belonging.

6.6 Mental Health Promotion and Education

Community-based mental health care also encompasses mental health promotion and education initiatives. These initiatives aim to raise awareness, reduce stigma, and foster mental health literacy within the community.

Mental health promotion activities may include awareness campaigns, workshops, and community events that focus on topics such as stress management, resilience-building, and self-care. Education programs aim to equip individuals with knowledge and skills to identify early signs of mental health disorders, seek help, and support others in their communities.

In Chapter 6, we have explored the importance of community-based mental health care in Ireland. Through the integration of mental health services with primary care, the provision of support through community mental health teams, home-based and outreach services, peer support groups, and mental health promotion initiatives, community-based care promotes accessibility, continuity, and social inclusion. By addressing mental health needs within the context of individuals' communities, Ireland's mental health system aims to improve overall well-being and enhance recovery outcomes.

Chapter 7: Challenges and Opportunities in Irish Mental Health Services

7.1 Introduction

While the mental health system in Ireland has made significant strides in recent years, there are still challenges that need to be addressed. This chapter explores some of the key challenges faced by mental health services in Ireland, as well as the opportunities for improvement and growth.

7.2 Insufficient Funding and Resources

One of the primary challenges in Irish mental health services is the issue of insufficient funding and resources. Despite increased recognition of the importance of mental health, funding levels often fall short of the actual needs of the population. This can result in long waiting lists, limited access to specialized services, and inadequate staffing levels.

To overcome this challenge, it is crucial to advocate for increased funding for mental health services and allocate resources effectively. Investing in mental health not only benefits individuals but also has a positive impact on society as a whole, reducing the burden on other sectors such as healthcare, criminal justice, and social welfare.

7.3 Stigma and Discrimination

Stigma and discrimination surrounding mental health remain significant barriers to care and support in Ireland.

Negative attitudes and misconceptions can prevent individuals from seeking help, lead to social isolation, and hinder the integration of individuals with mental health conditions into society.

Addressing stigma and discrimination requires a comprehensive approach that involves education, awareness campaigns, and challenging societal perceptions.

Promoting open conversations, sharing personal stories, and involving people with lived experience in mental health advocacy can help break down barriers and foster a more inclusive and supportive society.

7.4 Integration and Continuity of Care

Achieving seamless integration and continuity of care between different levels and sectors of mental health services is an ongoing challenge. Fragmentation can occur when individuals transition between primary care, community services, and specialized care, leading to gaps in treatment and a lack of coordination.

Efforts should be made to improve communication, collaboration, and information sharing among mental health professionals, primary care providers, and community supports. Integrated care models, care pathways, and shared electronic health records can facilitate a more coordinated approach and ensure individuals receive comprehensive and continuous support throughout their mental health journey.

7.5 Workforce Shortages and Training Needs

Workforce shortages and training needs pose significant challenges to the mental health system in Ireland. There is a shortage of mental health professionals, including psychiatrists, psychologists, nurses, and social workers, which can impact service delivery and access to care.

To address this challenge, it is essential to invest in mental health workforce development, including recruitment, training, and retention strategies.

Providing incentives for mental health professionals to work in underserved areas, offering specialized training programs, and promoting interdisciplinary collaboration can help build a strong and sustainable mental health workforce.

7.6 Digital Mental Health and Technology

Advancements in technology present both challenges and opportunities for mental health services in Ireland. The rapid expansion of digital mental health interventions, such as telehealth and smartphone applications, has the potential to enhance access to care, improve monitoring and self-management, and overcome geographical barriers.

However, challenges related to privacy, data security, and equitable access to technology must be addressed. It is crucial to ensure that digital mental health interventions are evidence-based, culturally appropriate, and integrated into existing service frameworks. Combining the advantages of technology with personalized, human-centered care can lead to more innovative and effective mental health services.

7.7 Opportunities for Innovation and Collaboration

Despite the challenges, there are opportunities for innovation and collaboration within Irish mental health services. Engaging with service users, their families, and community organizations can lead to co-designing services that meet the diverse needs of individuals.

Exploring partnerships with academic institutions, research organizations, and technology companies can foster innovation in mental health interventions and service delivery models. Embracing research and evidence-based practices, along with continuous evaluation and quality improvement, can further enhance the effectiveness and efficiency of mental health services in Ireland.

In Chapter 7, we have highlighted some of the key challenges and opportunities in Irish mental health services.

By addressing funding and resource issues, combating stigma, improving integration and continuity of care, addressing workforce shortages, harnessing the potential of technology, and fostering collaboration and innovation, the mental health system in Ireland can continue to evolve and provide high-quality care that meets the diverse needs of its population.

Chapter 8: Advocacy and Empowerment for Mental Health Specialists

8.1 The Role of Advocacy in Mental Health

Advocacy plays a crucial role in promoting the rights, well-being, and professional development of mental health specialists. It involves actively speaking up and working towards positive change in policies, practices, and public attitudes related to mental health. In this chapter, we explore the importance of advocacy and empowerment for mental health specialists in Ireland.

8.2 Professional Organizations and Associations

Professional organizations and associations play a significant role in advocating for the rights and interests of mental health specialists. These organizations provide a platform for professionals to come together, share knowledge, collaborate, and collectively address challenges faced in the field.

In Ireland, mental health professionals can join organizations such as the Irish Association of Counselling and Psychotherapy (IACP), the Irish Psychiatric Association (IPA), and the Psychological Society of Ireland (PSI). These organizations advocate for professional standards, ethical guidelines, and the recognition of mental health professionals' expertise. They also provide resources, continuing education opportunities, and support networks for mental health specialists.

8.3 Promoting Professional Well-being and Self-Care

Advocacy for mental health specialists includes promoting their own professional well-being and self-care. The demanding nature of the work can lead to burnout, compassion fatigue, and emotional exhaustion. It is essential for mental health professionals to prioritize self-care, establish healthy boundaries, and seek support when needed.

Advocacy efforts should focus on creating a supportive work environment, promoting work-life balance, and providing resources for mental health professionals' self-care.

This can include access to supervision, peer support, training on resilience-building, and opportunities for professional development and career advancement.

8.4 Continuing Education and Professional Development

Advocacy and empowerment for mental health specialists involve ensuring access to quality continuing education and professional development opportunities. Staying updated on the latest research, best practices, and emerging treatment modalities is crucial for delivering effective and evidence-based care.

Advocacy efforts should aim to secure funding for professional development programs, workshops, conferences, and training opportunities. Collaborations between professional organizations, academic institutions, and mental health services can facilitate the dissemination of knowledge and the enhancement of professional competencies.

8.5 Workforce Support and Recognition

Advocacy for mental health specialists includes advocating for appropriate workforce support, recognition, and remuneration. Mental health professionals should be provided with a supportive work environment, reasonable caseloads, and adequate resources to deliver quality care.

Advocacy efforts should focus on promoting fair compensation, career progression opportunities, and recognition of mental health professionals' contributions to the field.

This can involve engaging with policymakers, negotiating for improved working conditions, and participating in workforce planning initiatives.

8.6 Influencing Mental Health Policies and Legislation

Advocacy for mental health specialists extends to influencing mental health policies and legislation at the national level. Mental health professionals have first-hand knowledge of the challenges faced by individuals with mental health conditions and the gaps in service provision.

By engaging in policy discussions, participating in consultations, and providing expert input, mental health specialists can contribute to the development of policies that prioritize prevention, early intervention, and comprehensive mental health care. Advocacy efforts should aim to ensure that mental health policies align with international best practices, promote human rights, and address the specific needs of the Irish population.

8.7 Reducing Stigma and Promoting Public Awareness

Advocacy for mental health specialists involves actively working towards reducing stigma and promoting public awareness of mental health issues. By challenging misconceptions, engaging in public campaigns, and sharing personal stories, mental health professionals can contribute to changing societal attitudes towards mental health.

Advocacy efforts should focus on education programs in schools, workplaces, and communities to promote mental health literacy, early intervention, and DE stigmatization. Collaboration with media outlets, community organizations, and advocacy groups can amplify the voices of mental health specialists and raise public awareness.

In Chapter 8, we have explored the importance of advocacy and empowerment for mental health specialists in Ireland. By actively engaging in advocacy efforts, mental health specialists can contribute to shaping policies, promoting professional well-being, influencing public perception, and creating a supportive environment for themselves and their colleagues. By working together and leveraging their expertise, mental health specialists can bring about positive change in the mental health sector and improve outcomes for individuals with mental health conditions.

Chapter 9: Understanding Mental Health Tribunals

9.1 The Mental Health Commission:

The Mental Health Commission in Ireland plays a vital role in overseeing and regulating mental health services to ensure the highest standards of care and protection for individuals experiencing mental health challenges. As an independent statutory body, the Commission functions as an authoritative voice in the mental health sector, working collaboratively with various stakeholders including healthcare providers, policymakers, and service users.

The Commission's responsibilities encompass monitoring and inspecting mental health services, promoting quality improvement initiatives, enforcing regulatory compliance, and advocating for the rights and well-being of patients.

By establishing standards, conducting inspections, and offering guidance, the Mental Health Commission aims to create a more transparent, accountable, and person-centred mental health system in Ireland.

9.2 The Mental Health Act 2001 is an important piece of legislation in Ireland that governs the rights, care, and treatment of individuals with mental health disorders. Here are some key provisions of the Mental Health Act 2001:

1. Definition of Mental Disorder: The Act defines a mental disorder as a condition that affects the mind, including mental illness, mental impairment, or severe personality disorder.

2. Involuntary Admission: The Act establishes procedures for the involuntary admission of individuals to approved psychiatric centres. It outlines criteria for admission, such as the presence of a mental disorder, the need for treatment, and the risk to the person's health or safety.

3. Voluntary Admission: The Act also provides for voluntary admission to psychiatric centres, allowing individuals to seek treatment and care for their mental health issues voluntarily.

4. Independent Review of Detention: The Act
    establishes the Mental Health Commission, which
    is responsible for reviewing and monitoring the
    detention and care of individuals in approved
    centres. The Commission oversees the rights and
    welfare of patients, ensuring that they receive
    appropriate care and treatment.

5. Rights of Detained Persons: The Act specifies the
    rights of detained individuals, including the right to
    be informed about their admission, access to legal
    representation, the right to communicate with
    others, and the right to challenge their detention
    through a Mental Health Tribunal.

6. Mental Health Tribunals: The Act establishes
    Mental Health Tribunals, which are independent
    bodies responsible for reviewing the detention of
    individuals in approved centres. The tribunals
    assess the necessity and appropriateness of
    continued detention and can make decisions
    regarding release or conditions of care.

7. Consent and Capacity: The Act addresses issues of
    consent and capacity in mental health treatment. It
    outlines provisions for assessing a person's capacity
    to consent to treatment and establishes safeguards
    to ensure that decisions are made in the person's
    best interests.

8. Advance Healthcare Directives: The Act allows individuals to create Advance Healthcare Directives, which specify their preferences regarding treatment and care in the event of a future loss of capacity to make decisions.

9. Advocacy and Support: The Act recognizes the importance of advocacy and support for individuals with mental health disorders. It provides for the appointment of designated representatives who can support and represent the interests of patients.

These are some of the key provisions of the Mental Health Act 2001 in Ireland. It's important to refer to the complete Act for a comprehensive understanding of its content, including any subsequent amendments or regulations that may have been made since its enactment.

9.3 What are the criteria for involuntary admission?

In Ireland, the criteria for involuntary admission to a psychiatric centre are outlined in the Mental Health Act 2001.

These criteria serve as a legal framework to ensure that individuals with severe mental health disorders receive the necessary care and treatment. The criteria for involuntary admission typically include the following elements:

1. Mental Disorder: The individual must have a mental disorder, which is defined as a condition that affects the mind, including mental illness, mental impairment, or severe personality disorder.

The disorder should be of a nature and degree that warrants admission to a psychiatric centre.

2. Need for Treatment: The person's mental disorder must be such that they require treatment in their own best interest or for the protection of others. The treatment should address the person's mental health needs, alleviate their symptoms, or prevent a deterioration of their condition.

3. Risk to Health or Safety: There must be a risk to the person's health or safety if they do not receive treatment. This risk can be assessed based on the person's behaviour, symptoms, and the potential harm they may pose to themselves or others.

It's important to note that the decision for involuntary admission is not taken lightly, and the criteria are designed to balance the rights of the individual with the need to ensure their well-being and safety. The assessment and decision regarding involuntary admission are typically made by healthcare professionals, often in consultation with an approved medical officer, who assesses the person's condition and determines whether the criteria for admission are met.

9.4 Purpose and Function of Mental Health Tribunal Panels: Mental health tribunal panels are a crucial component of the MHC's work. These panels review the detention of individuals in psychiatric centres and make decisions regarding their continued detention or release.

Laypersons on tribunal panels provide an impartial and informed perspective, ensuring that the rights and interests of patients are respected and protected. As a lay advocate, you have the responsibility to assess the appropriateness of the individual's detention and contribute to decision-making.

A tribunal panel typically consists of the following personnel:

1. Chairperson: The chairperson is responsible for overseeing the proceedings and ensuring that they are conducted in a fair and impartial manner. They will either be a qualified solicitor or barrister and are familiar with the relevant legislation and regulations.

2. Medical Member: The medical member is usually a qualified psychiatrist. Their role is to provide a clinical perspective, assess the patient's condition, and contribute to the decision-making process based on their medical knowledge and experience.

3. Layperson: The layperson, is a non-professional member of the panel who represents the broader community and brings an independent perspective. They do not have a professional background in mental health but offer insights into the social, cultural, and personal aspects of the patient's situation. The layperson ensures that the patient's rights and interests are considered and may advocate for alternative perspectives or approaches.

Patient's legal representation

In the context of a tribunal panel, the patient has the right to legal representation. Legal representation ensures that the patient's interests are adequately represented and their rights are protected throughout the tribunal process.

The role of legal representation may include:

1. Advising the patient: The legal representative provides guidance and advice to the patient regarding their rights, legal options, and the tribunal process. They help the patient understand the implications of their choices and make informed decisions.

2. Preparing the case: The legal representative assists in gathering relevant information, preparing evidence, and presenting a case on behalf of the patient. They may review medical records, interview witnesses, and consult with experts to build a strong argument.

3. Advocacy during the hearing: The legal representative presents the patient's case before the tribunal panel, cross-examines witnesses, and challenges evidence or arguments that are not in the patient's favour. They ensure that the patient's voice is heard and their rights are protected.

4. Legal analysis and submissions: The legal representative analyses the legal aspects of the case, applies relevant laws and regulations, and makes legal submissions to support the patient's position. They may argue for the patient's release, review of treatment plans, or other necessary legal actions.

5. Ensuring procedural fairness: The legal representative ensures that the tribunal proceedings adhere to the principles of procedural fairness and that the patient's rights are respected. They may object to any unfair procedures, biased decisions, or breaches of legal requirements.

Also, the treating consultant psychiatrist is in attendance to discuss the patient's current diagnosis and progress to date and answer questions put to them in relation to the patient.

9.5 Legal Framework and Key Legislation: Mental health tribunals operate within a legal framework governed by the Mental Health Act and other relevant legislation. These laws outline the rights and protections afforded to individuals experiencing mental health challenges. For example, the Mental Health Act 2001 establishes the criteria for involuntary admission and detention, while the Assisted Decision-Making (Capacity) Act 2015 provides guidance on assessing capacity and respecting individuals' autonomy.

9.6 The Importance of Laypersons in Tribunal Panels: Laypersons bring a valuable perspective to tribunal panels by representing the wider community and offering an independent viewpoint. By participating in hearings, laypersons ensure that the decisions made reflect a balanced consideration of the patient's best interests. For instance, as a layperson, you may contribute insights into the potential impact of detention on an individual's social and family life, providing a holistic understanding of their circumstances.

9.7 Ethical Considerations and Confidentiality: Laypersons must adhere to ethical principles, maintaining confidentiality and respecting the privacy of patients. This includes handling sensitive information appropriately and ensuring that discussions during tribunal hearings remain confidential. Ethical dilemmas may arise, such as balancing the patient's right to autonomy with the need for protection.

For instance, you might encounter situations where a patient's refusal of treatment raises concerns about their well-being, necessitating careful consideration and consultation with healthcare professionals.

Conclusion: Understanding the workings of mental health tribunals is paramount for effective advocacy within psychiatric wards.

As a layperson working for the Mental Health Commission, your role on tribunal panels contributes to safeguarding the rights and well-being of individuals experiencing mental health challenges.

Embracing the significance of the Mental Health Commission's oversight and the legal framework governing tribunal proceedings allows you to approach your responsibilities with clarity and purpose. By fulfilling your role impartially and collaborating with healthcare professionals, you can ensure a fair and just decision-making process that upholds the dignity and rights of those you serve.

Chapter 10: The Layperson's Role

10.1 Qualities and Skills of an Effective Lay Person: Effective lay people possess qualities such as empathy, active listening, and the ability to communicate clearly and compassionately.

These skills allow you to connect with patients, understand their perspectives, and advocate for their rights.

For example, active listening helps you to truly comprehend a patient's experiences and concerns, enabling you to convey their viewpoints accurately during tribunal proceedings.

10.2 Working Collaboratively with Healthcare Professionals: Collaboration with healthcare professionals is essential for effective advocacy. Developing constructive relationships with psychiatrists, nurses, and other professionals fosters a team-based approach to patient care.

By actively participating in discussions and sharing insights from the layperson's perspective, you contribute to a comprehensive understanding of the patient's situation. For instance, your input may shed light on the patient's social support system or their community resources, which can inform the decision-making process and potential alternatives to detention.

10.3 Cultural Sensitivity and Diversity Awareness: Cultural sensitivity is crucial in advocating for individuals from diverse backgrounds. Recognizing and respecting cultural differences helps ensure that the rights and needs of all patients are acknowledged. For example, understanding cultural beliefs and practices related to mental health can contribute to more effective communication and decision-making. It's important to approach each patient with an open mind and willingness to learn about their unique cultural experiences.

10.4 Confidentiality and Maintaining Boundaries: As a lay advocate, you must maintain strict confidentiality and respect the privacy of patients. This includes handling personal information and case details discreetly, both during and outside of tribunal proceedings. Respecting professional boundaries is essential to establish trust and ensure ethical practice. For instance, refraining from discussing specific cases or patient details outside of the necessary professional contexts demonstrates your commitment to maintaining confidentiality.

10.5 Building Rapport and Effective Communication: Building rapport with patients is essential for being an effective layperson.

Establishing a trusting and respectful relationship helps patients feel comfortable sharing their experiences and concerns. Effective communication techniques, such as using plain language, active listening, and empathy, can facilitate productive interactions. For example, paraphrasing and summarizing a patient's statements during a tribunal hearing can demonstrate that their voice is being heard and understood.

Conclusion: As a lay advocate, your qualities and skills play a pivotal role in supporting patients throughout the tribunal process. Your empathetic approach, effective communication, and cultural sensitivity enable you to connect with patients and understand their unique experiences. Collaborating with healthcare professionals while maintaining your independent perspective enhances the interdisciplinary approach to patient care.

Upholding confidentiality, setting boundaries, and building rapport contribute to a trusting relationship with patients, empowering them to express their views and participate actively in the decision-making process.

As you continue to embrace your role as a layperson, remember that your advocacy efforts bring valuable insights and balance to mental health tribunal panels.

Chapter 11: The Tribunal Process

11.1 Preparing for Tribunal Hearings: Thorough preparation is key to participating effectively in tribunal hearings. This includes reviewing relevant documentation, familiarizing yourself with the patient's case history, and identifying key points for discussion.

Additionally, understanding the tribunal's procedural rules and guidelines ensures that hearings are conducted fairly and in accordance with legal requirements. For instance, reviewing previous tribunal decisions can provide valuable insights into precedents and considerations.

11.2 Understanding Patients' Rights: A comprehensive understanding of patients' rights is crucial for advocating on their behalf during tribunal proceedings. This includes rights such as informed consent, access to information, and the right to be heard. Familiarizing yourself with these rights ensures that you can raise relevant concerns and contribute to fair decision-making. For example, understanding a patient's right to challenge their detention and the criteria for release can inform your arguments and recommendations.

11.3 Conducting Fair and Impartial Hearings: As a layperson, your role is to contribute to fair and impartial hearings. This requires actively listening to all parties involved, considering different perspectives, and asking relevant questions to clarify information. Fairness also means ensuring that the patient has the opportunity to express their views and concerns. For instance, providing a supportive environment for the patient to share their experiences can help the tribunal panel gain a comprehensive understanding of their circumstances.

11.4 Decision-Making and Providing Recommendations: After considering all the relevant information presented during the hearing, the tribunal panel must make decisions regarding the patient's detention or release.

Your role as a lay advocate is to contribute to this decision-making process by offering informed recommendations based on the patient's best interests and their rights. For example, you might recommend a review of the treatment plan, exploring community-based support options, or additional safeguards to protect the patient's well-being.

11.5 Documenting Proceedings and Writing Reports: Accurate and detailed documentation is essential for maintaining transparency and accountability. Throughout the tribunal process, it is important to document key discussions, decisions, and any dissenting opinions. After the hearing, a comprehensive report should be prepared that outlines the panel's findings and recommendations. Your contributions to these reports can help ensure that the patient's concerns and rights are accurately represented.

Conclusion: Navigating the tribunal process effectively requires thorough preparation, a comprehensive understanding of patients' rights, and a commitment to conducting fair and impartial hearings. Your role as a lay advocate involves assessing patients' circumstances and contributing informed recommendations to the decision-making process. Documenting proceedings accurately and writing comprehensive reports are essential for transparency and accountability.

By adhering to procedural rules and ethical considerations, you contribute to a tribunal process that respects patients' dignity, upholds their rights, and strives for the best possible outcomes in their mental health care journey.

Chapter 12: Mental Health and the Law

12.1 Mental Health Act and Relevant Legislation: Understanding the Mental Health Act and other relevant legislation is crucial for navigating the legal aspects of tribunal panels. This includes familiarizing yourself with the provisions related to involuntary admission, and detention criteria. For example, understanding the criteria for detention can help you assess whether the patient's detention is justified and compliant with legal requirements.

12.2 Involuntary Admission and Detention Criteria: Exploring the criteria for involuntary admission and detention is essential for assessing the appropriateness of a patient's current status.

Understanding the legal requirements for admission, such as the presence of a mental disorder and the risk to the patient's health or safety, enables you to contribute to the decision-making process. For instance, you might question the necessity of continued detention if the patient's condition has improved and no longer meets the criteria.

12.3 Consent and Capacity Assessment: The issue of consent and capacity is significant when it comes to mental health treatment and detention. Understanding the legal principles and assessment processes related to capacity ensures that patients' autonomy and decision-making rights are respected.

12.4 Challenging Detention and Advocating for Alternatives: Occasionally, it may be necessary to challenge the legality of a patient's detention or advocate for alternative forms of care and support. Understanding the legal mechanisms for challenging detention and exploring alternatives, such as supported housing, is essential for advocating in the best interests of the patient. For example, you might gather evidence to support a request for a review of the detention or propose less restrictive alternatives that prioritize the patient's well-being as the hearing progresses.

Conclusion: A deep understanding of the Mental Health Act 2001 and other relevant legislation empowers you to navigate the legal aspects of mental health tribunal panels with confidence. Recognizing the criteria for involuntary admission, the principles of consent and capacity, and the role of mental health review boards enables you to advocate effectively for patients' rights and well-being. Your familiarity with legal provisions related to challenging detention and advocating for alternatives strengthens your ability to ensure the least restrictive measures are pursued in patients' best interests. As you engage with the legal framework, your advocacy efforts contribute to a just and rights-based mental health system.

Chapter 13: Addressing Ethical Dilemmas

13.1 Balancing Autonomy and Protection: Ethical dilemmas often arise when balancing a patient's autonomy and the need for protection. Recognizing and addressing these dilemmas is crucial for advocating effectively.

For instance, when a patient refuses treatment that may be necessary for their well-being, you might collaborate with healthcare professionals to explore less restrictive interventions while respecting the patient's autonomy.

13.2 Coercion and Least Restrictive Measures: Advocating for the least restrictive measures possible is an ethical principle that guides decision-making. Working with healthcare professionals, you can advocate for alternatives to detention or treatments that minimize coercion.

For example, you might propose therapeutic interventions that allow the patient to maintain their independence while addressing their mental health needs.

13.3 Capacity Assessment and Informed Consent: Capacity assessment and informed consent are critical considerations in the tribunal process.

Ensuring that patients have the capacity to understand the implications of their decisions and provide informed consent is paramount. As a layperson, you might collaborate with healthcare professionals to assess capacity accurately and advocate for procedures that prioritize patients' understanding and involvement in their treatment decisions.

13.4 Supporting Patients: Decision-Making Process Respecting and supporting patients' decision-making process is essential for ethical advocacy. This includes providing them with relevant information, ensuring comprehension, and facilitating their involvement in decision-making.

For example, you might collaborate with healthcare professionals to present information in a manner that the patient can understand and explore shared decision-making approaches that empower the patient to actively participate in determining their treatment plan or discharge plan.

13.5 Confidentiality and Privacy: Maintaining confidentiality and respecting patients' privacy are fundamental ethical principles. As a layperson, you must handle sensitive patient information with care and ensure that it is shared only with authorized individuals involved in the tribunal process. Respecting privacy and confidentiality helps build trust with patients and ensures the integrity of the advocacy process.

13.6 Dual Roles and Conflicts of Interest: It is crucial to identify and manage any potential conflicts of interest that may arise from your role as a layperson.

Dual roles, such as having personal or professional relationships with patients or healthcare professionals, can present ethical challenges. Recognizing and appropriately addressing conflicts of interest helps maintain the integrity and impartiality of the advocacy process.

13.7 Self-Care and Boundaries: Engaging in mental health advocacy can be emotionally demanding. Practicing self-care and setting boundaries are essential for maintaining your well-being and ensuring effective advocacy.

Taking breaks, seeking support, and engaging in reflective practices help prevent burnout and ensure that you can continue to provide compassionate and objective advocacy for patients.

Addressing ethical dilemmas is an essential aspect of your role as a layperson on mental health tribunal panels. Striking a balance between autonomy and protection, advocating for the least restrictive measures, and ensuring capacity assessment and informed consent reflect your commitment to ethical advocacy. Upholding confidentiality, recognizing conflicts of interest, and practicing self-care promote ethical conduct and maintain the integrity of the advocacy process. Your dedication to ethical principles ensures that patients receive compassionate and respectful care, and their rights are upheld throughout the tribunal process.

Conclusion:

As a layperson working for the Mental Health Commission in Ireland, you play a crucial role in safeguarding the rights and well-being of individuals within psychiatric wards. Your understanding of mental health tribunals, your qualities as an effective lay advocate, and your knowledge of the legal framework and ethical considerations contribute to fair and compassionate decision-making. By upholding the principles of autonomy, dignity, and justice, you contribute to a mental health system that respects the diversity and rights of those you serve.

Your commitment to continuous learning and self-care enables you to make a meaningful impact on the lives of individuals experiencing mental health challenges, creating a more compassionate and inclusive mental health system in Ireland.

The field of mental health services in Ireland is continually evolving, driven by a growing recognition of the importance of mental health and the need for comprehensive care and support. Throughout this book, we have explored various aspects of mental health services from the perspective of a mental health specialist. We have delved into understanding mental health, the overview of mental health services in Ireland, assessing and diagnosing mental health disorders, treatment approaches, specialized services, community-based care, challenges and opportunities, and the role of advocacy and empowerment.

Building a resilient mental health system requires a multi-faceted approach that addresses the needs of individuals, communities, and society as a whole.

It involves collaboration, innovation, and a commitment to continuous improvement. By integrating these key elements, Ireland can strive towards a mental health system that is responsive, accessible, and effective.

To build a resilient mental health system, it is essential to:

Invest in Mental Health: Adequate funding and resources are crucial to meet the increasing demand for mental health services.

By investing in mental health, Ireland can ensure the availability of a wide range of services, reduce waiting times, and provide comprehensive support to individuals across the lifespan.

Promote Prevention and Early Intervention: Emphasizing prevention and early intervention is vital for reducing the burden of mental health disorders. By implementing targeted prevention programs, raising awareness, and providing accessible early intervention services, Ireland can support individuals in maintaining good mental health and addressing issues before they escalate.

Foster Integration and Continuity of Care: Seamless integration and continuity of care are essential for individuals navigating the mental health system. Collaboration between primary care providers, community services, specialized care, and support networks is critical to ensure comprehensive and coordinated care throughout individuals' mental health journeys.

Address Stigma and Discrimination: Stigma and discrimination surrounding mental health persist as significant barriers to seeking help and receiving adequate support.

By challenging stereotypes, promoting education, and fostering a culture of acceptance and understanding, Ireland can create an environment that encourages individuals to seek help without fear of judgment or discrimination.

Enhance Workforce Development and Support: A well-trained and supported workforce is the backbone of a resilient mental health system. Investing in workforce development, providing ongoing training opportunities, and prioritizing mental health professionals' well-being can improve service delivery, reduce burnout, and attract and retain talented individuals in the field.

Embrace Technology and Innovation: The rapid advancement of technology presents opportunities to enhance mental health services. Integrating digital mental health interventions, telehealth, and electronic health records can increase accessibility, improve monitoring, and support self-management. However, careful attention must be given to privacy, security, and equitable access to ensure the benefits of technology reach all individuals.

Empower Individuals and Communities: Empowering individuals with mental health conditions and their communities is fundamental to building a resilient mental health system. Providing education, fostering self-advocacy skills, and involving individuals in decision-making processes can contribute to their overall well-being and sense of ownership over their recovery journey.

By embracing these principles and working together, mental health specialists, policymakers, communities, and individuals can contribute to the development of a resilient mental health system in Ireland. This system recognizes the diverse needs of individuals, promotes holistic care, and ensures that mental health is prioritized as a fundamental aspect of overall well-being.

Building a resilient mental health system is an ongoing journey, and it requires continuous collaboration, adaptation, and a shared commitment to supporting individuals on their path to mental wellness.

References:

Department of Health. (2018). Sharing the Vision: A Mental Health Policy for Everyone. Dublin, Ireland: Government of Ireland.

Mental Health Reform. (2021). Mental Health in Ireland: Facts and Figures. Retrieved from https://www.mentalhealthreform.ie/learn/facts-and-figures/

Irish Association of Counselling and Psychotherapy (IACP). (n.d.). Retrieved from https://iacp.ie/

Irish Psychiatric Association (IPA). (n.d.). Retrieved from https://www.irishpsychiatry.ie/

Psychological Society of Ireland (PSI). (n.d.). Retrieved from https://www.psihq.ie/

World Health Organization. (2021). Mental Health Atlas 2021. Geneva: World Health Organization.

Mental Health Commission. (2019). Quality Framework for Mental Health Services in Ireland. Dublin, Ireland: Mental Health Commission.

HSE National Office for Suicide Prevention. (2021). Connecting for Life: Ireland's National Strategy to Reduce Suicide 2015-2020. Dublin, Ireland: Health Service Executive.

O'Connor, R. C., & Pirkis, J. (2020). The International Handbook of Suicide Prevention (2nd ed.). John Wiley & Sons.

Barry, M. M., Clarke, A. M., Jenkins, R., & Patel, V. (Eds.). (2013). Implementing Mental Health Promotion. Springer. Mental Health Commission (Ireland). (n.d.). About the Mental Health Commission. Retrieved from https://www.mhcirl.ie/about-us/

Mental Health Act 2001. Retrieved from https://www.irishstatutebook.ie/eli/2001/act/25/enacted/en/print.html

Assisted Decision-Making (Capacity) Act 2015. Retrieved from https://www.irishstatutebook.ie/eli/2015/act/64/enacted/en/html

Department of Health (Ireland). (2019). Mental Health Policy A Vision for Change. Retrieved from https://www.gov.ie/en/publication/2317b-mental-health-policy-a-vision-for-change/

Mental Health Tribunal. (n.d.). What we do. Retrieved from https://www.mentalhealthtribunal.ie/en/about/what-we-do/

www.ingramcontent.com/pod-product-compliance
Lightning Source LLC
Chambersburg PA
CBHW050051260726
48658CB00005B/1890